Be Water, Be One©

An Introductory Guide to the New Book:

**"LifeForce – Just For the Health Of It!
A Guide to Better Living Through Natural Energy"©**

By:
Lee E. Gresser, M.D.
&
William Nusz

"*Empty your mind. Be formless, shapeless-like water. If you put water into a cup, it becomes the cup. If you put water into a bottle, it becomes the bottle. If you put it in a teapot, it becomes the teapot. Now, water can flow or it can crash. Be water, my friend!*" (*And be one with Air; be one with just Being!*)

Bruce Lee

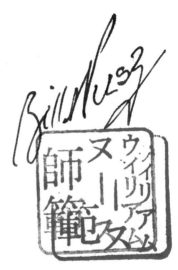

3

Be Water, Be One©
An Introductory Guide to the New Book:
LifeForce – Just For the Health of It!
A Guide to Better Living Through Natural Energy ©

ISBN: 0-9748645-0-1

This book is an introductory compliment to the
forthcoming book:

LIFEFORCE - Just For The Health of It!
A Guide to Better Living Through Natural Energy and a
complete guide to natural energy therapy and magnets --an
energy force that promises to revolutionize 21st-century
medicine.

‡ Fact references courtesy of National Institute of Health

For more information contact: bewater_beone@yahoo.com

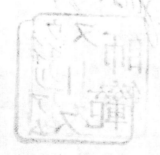

ABOUT THIS BOOK

In this and our forthcoming book, the history and science of natural energy is presented with several studies (1,2,3), including those by Michael I. Weintraub M.D. on repetitive wrist motion and numbness in the extremities. They show why natural energy sources, including magnets, have a significant role in helping to ease discomfort, assist with healing and promote a healthier state of well being.   To integrate eastern and western health and philosophy, the lifestyle and art of The Martial Arts was chosen as a means of introducing such a concept through William Nusz who is the trainer of the US Koshiki Karate Team. The martial arts have used natural energy for centuries to enhance the LifeForce and today's modern products enhance its training.

It is explained how and why sources of natural energy, including magnets, have been used as powerful healing tools for decades in Europe and Asia, as well as a well documented history of success that can be traced back thousands of years. Now, for the first time, is a comprehensive guide that discusses more than just magnets. This book will detail how you are part of the completely natural energy System that is the essence of Nature. The LIFEFORCE is the natural energy that exists within you and surrounds you constantly. What you want and need to know about natural energy therapy and magnets is in this introductory book and the forthcoming book **"Lifeforce-Just For The Health Of It!"**

While many other writers on this subject distract their readers with idiolect and jargon, I have provided you with a clear explanation of the basic principles and practices of natural energy therapy. This includes in-depth details on the use of magnets, and explanations on how natural energy can help overcome health problems, improve health and wellness and improve your quality of life. The recent discovery of magnetic receptors in the human brain has confirmed what the ancient Chinese, Indians, Egyptians, and Greeks always knew: that human beings are strongly influenced by the Earth's magnetic field, and that by subtly altering our own energy fields with magnets we can restore proper balance to our body systems. More than 200 million people in the United States and around the world have already successfully used this science of natural energy therapy.

Natural energy therapy, which is supported by a growing body of scientific evidence, is becoming increasingly popular in the United States. Used also by a growing number of professional athletes, natural energy therapy and magnets can help alleviate chronic discomfort or that associated with acute injuries. LIFEFORCE tells you what you need to know about this revolutionary approach to healing.

You will learn:

- Which sources of natural energy can help specific conditions
- How to use natural energy therapy in conjunction with other therapies
- The historical and scientific background of natural energy therapy
- How research into magnets and the use of natural energy therapy may affect the future of medicine

And much more!

6

Introductory Book Contents:

Prologue: My Legacy

PROLOGUE: My Legacy

After all my experience in medicine and health care, I have come to realize that I have a story to tell and a vast amount of knowledge to share with you about improving your quality of life. I feel the best way to achieve this effort is to do like in Olden times and sit down like a Grandfather storyteller and tell you all, plainly and simply, about an ancient system of healing arts that has greatly been ignored and hidden in the dark. *Like the Bardic poets of yesteryear, I will relate in plain, simple terms, sometimes taking liberties with grammar, as is often the case when talking in plain conversational English, the simple concept of LifeForce and all its related techniques and solutions to the complexities of life! As you read this booklet, think of the information related in this booklet as casual conversation rather then a scientific or medical essay*

After practicing Family Medicine for 32 years, I realized that there was more out there that academic medicine did not know than what they did know. I was part of that mindset long before I retired. The intelligentsia knows it. Some egos cannot admit it. Some of what I have seen is not written in textbooks. Science will explain it one day but perhaps not in my lifetime. Nevertheless, what I have learned will hopefully be passed on for generations to come so that our children and their children's children will benefit and make this world a better place. My friend, Sean Mactire, has been instrumental in encouraging me to share my experiences. With his advice and pen that has produced many books on journaling, he has been a great asset to me. Now I can continue to help even more people than I have been able to do previously, one person at a time, throughout my career in medicine.

Ten years before I retired, I was introduced to nutritional and herbal medicine and found them to be complementary to a comprehensive health program. Unfortunately, I was taught relatively little about nutrition in medical school.

I then realized the "placebo effect" was real and not really a placebo because of the mind/body connection that was stimulated by chemicals in the brain called endorphins, which increased on verbal-auditory suggestion and in turn caused positive bodily responses.

You will be surprised to know that a placebo effect can be as high as 50%! Therefore, if I suggest that your pain will improve with this "green capsule"(filled with sugar), your pain will lessen or you will sleep better in up to 50% of cases. Drugs can do the same thing, usually up to 60% of the time and if you use enough drugs you can be pain free and/or you can sleep—sometimes forever!

Eastern medicine is focused more on energy medicine than biochemical medicine. It is an area that unknowing Western doctors find difficult to accept and understand even when they are personally hurting and have blinders on because of their inherent weakness to admit that unfamiliar solutions are out there for them to take advantage. They should forget they are doctors and look at the situation as if they are the patients. Unfortunately, they are not taught or trained to appreciate these unknown forces and how they

10

could possibly affect the human body, which are both a biochemical and an energy being. The Lifeforce that I am addressing connects the energy of the Mind, Body, and Spirit and hopefully will merge Eastern and Western medicine so that healthcare practitioners will no longer have to say to their patients "There is nothing more that I can do for you and you will just have to live with it." Humbug! They may not know what else to do but others with different life experiences do; albeit not necessarily scientific nor supported by double blind prospective studies on which many academicians, who are close minded, hang their hat. Shame on them if they are unaccepting, even if it is safe without side effects and it helps their patients! Let their patients decide if they do not have a good answer or get another opinion. That is good medicine.

Medical journals, which are published through the financial support of advertising by pharmaceutical companies, would publish articles that downplay any alternatives to drugs. Despite editorial boards, even in prestigious peer reviewed medical journals, I have seen very poor articles that politically favor certain products for financial gain.

What I have come to realize after studying and reading different viewpoints and methods of healing is that there is no one right way to improve the quality of life and prolong life. The energy force within us and around us can be harnessed and utilized for good until we die. Did you ever wonder about the Mind/Body connection when one's spouse dies and the other soon follows? Grandmother tales speak of dying from a "broken heart". It is a break in the connection of the Lifeforce.

For years we have been able to measure an aura around a living organism with Kirlian photography, using a type of infrared photographic film that records reflected heat waves. Newer digital

11

cameras in the future will have the ability to measure such energy forces. Together, with new technology, these old energy forces, which include far infrared, will be harnessed, better understood, and will play an important role in the next century of modern integrative medicine. We have just begun to see the controlled warmth and rapid healing powers with far infrared joint wraps and comforters.

In this new series of upcoming books, my intent is to integrate Eastern and Western medicine and philosophy, or traditional and alternative medicine or I should really say complementary medicine since it complements rather than being an alternative. It is not meant to replace, only to enhance one another. How old is either? Do we really know which one is the "alternative"? Complementary modalities generally are for chronic problems while traditional antibiotics and other specific drugs for acute life threatening situations have their place. When there is an integrative mindset more people will be helped, especially those who do not want to take drugs or undergo surgery or need to take less medication because of a high side effect profile. I hope to provide western orientated health practitioners some new energy tools to help more people. I will attempt to have you become more interested in prevention and investing in your health so that disease, disability, and eventually death can be delayed for many years and allow you to have a better quality of life. In subsequent books, all sports and age categories will be addressed with practical techniques and products to improve performance, decrease recovery time, improve sleep, lessen discomfort, increase mobility, balance, strength, and energy, and eventually reach your goals to health and wellness.

Most people are raised in a six-sided box for protection and comfort. Most are afraid to climb out of the box. Too threatening! Independent thinkers and entrepreneurs take a chance and climb out to become successful, healthy, and wealthy. 95% stay in the box and may or may not be comfortable. Lifeforce will open the box with the sword to do "good". It will be up to you to hold onto the sword and climb out of the box. When you do, your Lifeforce will be with you because you already have it, and your family and friends have it and together it is additive, addictive, supportive, and ever so powerful. So, now let me get comfortable on my toadstool and I will tell you how to do these very simple, very easy things that will ease the process of your life twenty fold!

LEE E. GRESSER M.D.

A. Water, Being and Air

We all have heard the expression; "Go with the flow!" but very few people understand what that means, even though the expression is as common as taking a deep breath. In Life, three elements of Nature completely control everyday existence – Air, Water, and Being! No one can live without them yet they are the most totally ignored things in anyone's life. Everyone takes air for granted because they take breathing for granted. You do not pay attention to your breathing because it is just occurs automatically. You overlook the key fact that your breathing defines and controls how you live! Everyone ignores the water you absolutely need to drink, bathe in, and use. Finally, no one, including you, pays any attention to their own being, the state of your body, and the state of things around you. Like the great majority of people, you just exist, take everything truly important for granted, and ignore the essentials of Life. Most people do not LIVE, they just function.. Again, you ignore the vital importance of water and being because these are just things that are there, things that just exist! And again, you forget that your being, and the water and air you use, defines your life and controls how you live. They also control whether you live or not!

Water, Being, and Air are the Essential Elements of Life, each different in substance, but totally the same in nature. Water is Energy, a Force. Being is also Energy and so is Air. Moreover, the three together are the foundation of Life - The LifeForce. Thus Water, Air, and Being are the essence of everything in nature and natural energy. In addition, the quality of and the amount of LifeForce you use in your life totally controls how well and how long you live.

Life is a challenge that most people think they have little control over, but True Living (living a good quality of life) is a martial art. That, by its very nature, is a ritual practice where the you must not only examine the issues of life or death but the nature of the self, defining and controlling how well and how long you will live. By completely embracing The LifeForce as a Path, a Way of Better Living, you become an essential one with Nature! Moreover, this So Easy, as Easy as BREATHING EASY, DRINKING LOTS OF GOOD WATER and JUST BEING! (Being at ease with all the things in your life! Being is the Whole Body Experience, which includes exercise and nutrition.) This is what it means to "GO WITH THE FLOW", because when you go with the flow, YOU ARE WATER, YOU ARE AIR, YOU ARE BEING! All together, you are BEING AS WATER!

Detach and relax! People stress over relaxing. So, do not think about it! Just be like water and just flow! This is how natural energy works for you and with you. Moreover, if you think of natural energy as if it is water that surrounds you every moment, you are like a boat on the water. You just float and flow with what is natural.

B. What Is LifeForce?

There is nothing paranormal, supernatural, or "alternative" about the use of natural energy products and techniques. It is all about using what is truly normal and natural in order to restore balance to the body and provide a means to developing and maintaining a better quality of life.

While it may appear that using natural energy is an "alternative health" practice, the true purpose is to bring a superior balance and awaken the subtle energies of the body, along with the fundamental energy within every human being, which is your LIFEFORCE.

Our goal is to introduce you to something that is a part of your life, but regrettably taken for granted. While many sources talk about "natural energy" the information is still very vague and never offers a plain explanation for everyone to understand. As a result, there are a number of wide spread misconceptions about what "natural energy" really is. Learning about LIFEFORCE is not totally meant to offer a system just for health and relaxation. This is just one part of a system that will provide you with the means to live a better quality of life.

Your body has seven principal energy centers and many secondary ones. As you learn more about LIFEFORCE and make the practice of using it more of your everyday routine, the specific configuration taken by your LIFEFORCE centers creates a connection to the corresponding subtle energies from Nature and your environment through a process of "wellness".

Now this sounds complex, but the daily practice of "wellness" is as simple as taking a shower, drinking a glass of water, and breathing. There is no mystery or mysticism to this simple, but very extraordinary means of improving your overall quality of life. All you are going to learn from this book is a better way to be healthy, wealthy and wise, using what Nature gave you and making better use of the resources that abound in you, and in Nature.

Every day you get up and spend your waking hours maneuvering down the same path trying to get to somewhere that you may not like once you do reach that point. LIFEFORCE is about "flow", about moving with life in a way that a boat sails on water, and it is about gaining a better understanding of the energy within your body and using it to make a difference in the lives you touch.

In addition, the Wellness Process provides you with the boat and the knowledge of how to enrich your life through the better use of your own energy and the energy around you. You also become more empowered by attaining a new ability to flow through life to a better living and better way of being, and you gain the ability to improve your life while you are asleep.

It is a Sunday ride in the park, 24/7, 365 days a year. So let us take the next step in learning what LIFEFORCE is and how the Wellness Process will enrich and empower you.

C. The LifeForce and Wellness

One all-encompassing driving LifeForce influences the destiny of the universe. An energy field generated by all living things, the LifeForce surrounds and penetrates everything, binding the universe together. Universal balance - life and death, creation and destruction - is reflected in the LifeForce, and thus is reflected from the LifeForce back into the universe at large. The LifeForce, for all the mystery and power it provides, is as much a part of the natural order as suns and planets and life itself.

The LifeForce has as many mysteries as it has aspects. It may be a non-feeling energy field, the sum of all creation. It may be an eternal entity, knowing, and unknowable. It may be both of these and more; it may be something else entirely. The only certain truth is that the LifeForce exists and is omnipresent, and that is enough for most who study its various influences. This somewhat enigmatic energy field consists of a multitude of properties.

The entire fabric of space is filled with the universal energy we call the LifeForce. It is vibrant and alive, existing everywhere and through everything. It both is the Tao yet transcends it, and contains the elements of ki, chi, prana, and spiritual Energy. With every breath, with every thought, heartbeat, and movement, the LifeForce is present. Vibrant and radiant, bursting with life and energy, this huge untapped reservoir of energy is what we call the LifeForce. When accepted as the valuable ally it is, the LifeForce can move with us, surround and penetrate us to the very core of being, and together move with us when we accept the inherent Will of the LifeForce to remove the blockages in life that prevent its full release in the matter cosmos.

The LifeForce is an essential part of nature --- like water --- it is a part of life itself; asking if it controls or can be controlled. It is like asking if a person controls his component cells or if they control him.

The LifeForce is both a tangible and intangible presence in life: an energy that exists in, through and around us and is the very essence of life itself.

The concept of ki - a concept of natural energy well known in the martial arts field for centuries- , is noted as the living force, in that Ki -the vital force of the body - the ki of a person can be drawn in increasing amount from the universe. In practice, ki is directed before body movement takes place.

A typical Energy-Body workshop begins with the assumption that "a field of energy exists in and around each human body". This energy is ki, "a single manifestation that includes emanations that can be measured by our present science, plus other esoteric or metaphorical emanations". One of the exercises in such a workshop is "sensing the energy body" where partners stand with arms extending towards each other. When one 'feels' the energy from one's partner, one is asked to move apart to find out how far away one can still sense the energy connection.

The LifeForce also is one's "connection to all life, time, and space; newness; and energy". As it is written "It is possible for a liar or a cheat to use Aiki or any of other five attacks to responses and aim for a 'kill' or a 'win' over somebody who has made the mistake of attacking him. But strange things begin to happen to people who become involved with Attack-tics ... even the most mean spirited of people begin to relinquish their grasp on their aggression, lose their anger, and reconnect with the living force".

The LifeForce is not the Cause, but the Effect - the universal energy. The LifeForce is energy that is freely given to all, like clay, to use or not to use. It is up to each of us to mold that clay, and through that molding, we decide what creation we construct with the energy, and to what end it serves. The LifeForce is a vehicle, which we can both manipulate and come to the ultimate decision on where the soul wishes to go (destiny). The LifeForce is the Ultimate energy that permeates the Universe.

In the physical universe, Energy is present in every atom that exists. The mental, emotional and spiritual quadrants also exist, yet at a much higher frequency than the matter cosmos, and simply because we cannot measure or monitor them accurately is not to say that they do not exist. They do exist. The Energy (which comprises the LifeForce, universal energy) that animates the Universe is neither good nor evil - it is unqualified until qualified by sentient beings, by you and I. The question of good and evil are questions of ethics, not of positively or negatively charged components of atomic matter.

Like a prism that bends the physical Energy rays of the Sun into a rainbow of colors, the purity of those colors depends upon the purity of the vessel radiating them. Purifying a vessel for the express purpose of coming up higher so that we on our own accord become the transparent vessel to radiate the Energy we were always meant to radiate (because that is our true destiny) means much more because WE chose it - not chosen for us by a superior deity - but of our own accord.

Wellness And Your Future Fate: As we see in the news everyday, tragedy befalls people when they least expect it. While a lot of these events seem out of anyone's control, such as being the victim of a terrorist attack, the majority of events in your life are totally in your control and how you interact with your environment and community will determine whether or not you become a victim of anything or whether or not your quality of life improves.

Life is fragile, but every person has the ability to build defenses that improve, protect, and prolong your life. This is the Fortress Formula of Wellness. Remember everything you do every moment of every day will have a positive or negative impact on your present and future quality of life. So NOT doing anything to help yourself is just as bad as DOING the wrong things that hurt, and shorten, your life.

The Fortress Formula Of Wellness - Every person in the world is born with a foundation of defenses that creates the beginnings of a Life Fortress that protects them from injury, illness, and other kinds of harm. This is your personal environment, and for the first years of life, the quality of this environment is based on the constructiveness or destructiveness of others. Therefore, by the time you are old enough to care for your own environment, your fortress is one of the three following types:

- The Wreck and Ruin
- The Basic Keep
- The Imperial Palace\

Even if your Fortress is a Ruin or at some point suffers the misfortune of becoming a Wreck, you can still create a Palace. All it takes is the TOOLS OF WELLNESS, which are key to building healthy walls that will allow you to enjoy all the benefits of Life:

22

- Physical Fitness
- Emotional Fitness
- Spiritual Fitness
- Coping Fitness - the mental tools (Stress Management Tools) that enable you to deal with all problems; the mental skills that help you interact with all types of people in a healthy manner; and the skills of mind and body to handle all levels of stress. This also includes Financial Management as a primary Stress Buster/Stress Control Tool.

This is something you cannot avoid, unless you like pain, stress and suffering. In order to achieve and live a better quality of life, you must make Wellness a part of your daily life. This means learning to Manage Stress, and learning to Manage the Things and People that cause Stress. Incorporating Wellness into your Life and creating a Wellness Lifestyle means learning to build your new home, your Palace, in a healthy, constructive way. Anyone can just throw a shelter together to get out of the rain, but that kind of inferior, careless structure will NEVER provide you with real protection. When the storms of Crisis and Pain hit you, you will be like the little pig in the house of straw. One blow and everything is Gone!

You can also run and hide, but you will not find any real protective shelter that way. If you like being a sitting duck, this option has a small bit of merit. Burying yourself in self-destructive activities - alcohol and drug abuse, overeating, reacting to people with anger or despair or isolation, etc. - is equally useless and unproductive. The result is just more pain and agony.

Building a Wellness Fortress does not mean you are creating a protective environment that isolates you from the world and the people in your life. You are just creating a state of being and a way of living. The armor of wellness is chain mail and breastplates of the mind and body; psychic body armor to shield you from the bullets of pain and stress that life shoots at you. It's a Spiritual Castle that makes the walls, floor and roof of your home a personal safe-haven; a stronghold of safety where you will always be to protect yourself and be comfortable, always sheltered from all the storms of life, yet able to let anyone enter your domain without fear of being harmed by them.

The benefit of creating a Wellness Fortress is that it helps you better manage stress and interact better with the people and things that are causing stress and pain (Stressors). Once you are in a position, in a state of being, that shows your ability to defend yourself, you soon learn from each encounter with stress and stressors that you are better and stronger then any of this stuff that once overwhelmed you with fear. You will also find yourself learning valuable things from these stressful people and things. You will discover that you can manage them better then you thought you could and you will learn that you have more power then these stressors.

A lot of people are unable to see the power they have or they are just afraid to use it. Then this weakness lets stress, stressors and other nasty things rule their lives and make them miserable. This is no way to live. So, in order to achieve a better quality of life, a Wellness Lifestyle, you have to see, know and use your power.

You also have to understand that fear is the enemy and it is always your fears that help create most of the damage that makes your life a wreck. Fear makes you powerless, but knowledge gives you power!   The more you learn about your stresses and fears, plus how to manage them, the more powerful you become.

Your LifeForce and your power are the foundation of your life and learning about LifeForce will teach you how fear and stress and stressors cause illness. It will also teach you how to protect yourself from harm and illness and how to use Wellness as a healing tool.

You will also discover that your Wellness Fortress is like an old-time castle. It is good old-fashioned REAL Magic, the reality of the true power of Mind and Body as One. Modern life has created very complex destructive problems that often cause some of the worst diseases and illnesses. But even though modern medical traditions and methods can produce results that in some past times could not have been achieved, many times miracles occur because of the use of older traditions and methods, along with the Power of Faith.

Ø Ø Ø

1. The Facts About Wellness And The Wellness Process

Wellness is health generating. A lack of well being in mind and body goes hand in hand with an impaired immune system, illness, shorter life, and increased medical expenditures. Scientists now can trace traffic along the nerve circuits in our brains and have begun to show how and where connections between attitudes and health take place. Strong indications are that the left and right prefrontal lobes of the brain are key sites that have these connections.

The Facts‡:

- Wellness oriented persons tend to have more activity in the brain's left prefrontal cortex when they respond to negative events, while anxious, pessimistic persons typically respond with activity in their right prefrontal lobes, and the activity tends to last longer than for happier persons.

- Those who react to stressful events with intense emotions have immune systems that are significantly weakened.

- This same lack of wellness can have profoundly different effects on different individuals. Those who have relatively large physiological reactions to the hassles, challenges, and frustrations of everyday life are at significantly higher risk for disease.

27

Many reports have linked emotional factors and health status, but precious little work has been dedicated to understanding the brain mechanisms by which wellness influences health.

So, by looking at brain circuitry and its outputs, you can get a handle on the mechanisms by which those outputs actually influence systemic bodily processes, like endocrine, immune, and autonomic functions, which play a role in modulating health.

People differ in the activation of their left and right prefrontal lobes of the cortex. Some people walk around on a daily basis with the left prefrontal region more activated. Others walk around with their right prefrontal regions more activated. The differences are consistent over time, and they correspond with certain personality traits, attitudes, and emotions. This is the "Wellness Difference", which is a matter of balance. The "balanced" person is wellness oriented and this is expressed in the manner in which they live their lives.

People with a more active left prefrontal region report themselves to be more cheerful, more enthusiastic, more eager, and alert, more engaged in life. They also show more persistence in pursuing their desired goals, and rapid recovery from negative life events.

There are also major physical differences in the immune systems. Persons who lack this wellness tendency respond to a stressful event with a more pronounced decline in immune function. Bottom-line is: They get sick faster and worse then others. These non-wellness people are also likely to have trouble turning off a negative emotion once it has turned on. They tend to be more vigilant for threats, hold on to negative life events, and take longer to recover from them.

Since this is an environmental problem, it can be controlled. Unfortunately, too many people turn to medications to control the damage caused by the lack of wellness structure in their lives. "Better living through chemistry" is the attitude. They do not realize that they can live better lives by adopting the attitude of "Better living through wellness ecology!"

Changing the emotional state of the individual to a positive state can control the entire system that generates stress responses in the brain. This is proof positive that there is something bi-directional about the system, that we can move it both up and down. The same stressful event can have profoundly different effects on different individuals, even widely different effects on the same individual in varying life circumstances.

More importantly, people who are non-wellness oriented, who show relatively large physiological responses to the hassles, and frustrations of everyday life are at significantly higher risk for disease. This is so even when their perceptions of the stress and their coping with it are present. Nevertheless, a change in environment and attitude can radically change your life. It is simply a matter of altering your "Life Ecology"! In addition, it is as easy as this

- Cultivate healthful behaviors - plenty of sleep, good nutrition, and exercise. Without those, you may get irritable reacting to things that should not and would not normally cause such reactions.

- Have a confidant, best friend, spouse, or someone else you can talk to honestly, to get support, feedback, and help putting events in perspective.

- Do not hold back emotional reactions. This does not mean go out and vent. This is   being hostile and its not productive. You want to be honest about the situation so you can deal with it effectively

- Get plenty of quality sleep.

- Drink lots of good quality water.

- In addition, think "Water". Adopt the attitude of being like water.

    You have to be mindful of your well-being and this calls for a huge lifestyle change, because what we are talking about is non-doing - how to be still. Moreover, this is something most adults do not do.

    Mindfulness is a life strategy technique that has very ancient roots. It is a way of living that is moment-to-moment, non-judgmental awareness. Most of the time the mind wants to be somewhere else, in the future, or in plans, or worry. All this may have little or nothing to do with the present reality. Gradually you train yourself to be more present in what is actually unfolding from moment to moment.

Ø Ø Ø

2. Pain

The one responsible for how your LifeForce acts and reacts to pain is you. If your LifeForce becomes overwhelmed by excessive pain, infection, or aging, then your health care provider shares in that responsibility.

Pain, one of the most common reasons for seeking medical care in the United States, is most commonly treated with medications. Frequently effective in the short term, they prove less so over longer periods. For patients with chronic pain, a host of Wellness Strategies© and alternatives can augment the effects of pain medication, often reducing the quantity needed or eliminating its use. Many strategies also can dramatically reduce disability related to pain, improve quality of life, and lower health care costs.

The Facts‡:

- More than 17 percent of U.S. patients seen by primary care physicians have persistent pain, according to the World Health Organization. Pain medications are the second most prescribed drugs (after cardiac-renal drugs) in visits to physicians' offices and emergency rooms.

- Chronic pain patients are at high risk for mental health disorders. In a study of male veterans with chronic low back pain, 32 percent had a history of depression, 65 percent had a history of alcohol use disorder, and 31 percent had a history of an anxiety disorder. According to a recent survey reported on the web site of the Johns Hopkins Center for Complementary and Alternative Medicine (CAM), which recently received a center grant sponsored by NIH, 40% of Americans use CAM for chronic conditions, most frequently for pain control. 50% used CAM because prescribed medications were ineffective. Over half of the patients used dietary supplements or herbal therapies and 2/3 found them to be helpful. 30-70% of cancer patients who are inadequately treated by their physicians turn to CAM in hopes of a cure or alleviation of their pain.

- A National Institutes of Health panel concluded that Wellness Strategies and other complimentary approaches, including the use of natural energy applications, relaxation training and cognitive/behavioral techniques help control pain in cancer, low back pain, arthritis, irritable bowel syndrome, headaches, and other medical conditions.

- Wellness resources can also help fight chronic pain. People who developed good wellness resource networking, including supportive family, often note less pain, use less pain medicine, and experience greater activity than those who have limited family support.

There's growing recognition that pain medication is often helpful in the short run, but for many people with persistent pain, pills and shots do not provide the total answer. Many times medications have side effects and people use them inconsistently, or do not use them at all.

Because Chronic Pain Management has become a specialty in itself, many general health professionals refer patients to these specialists because people in chronic pain are depressed and it takes time to ventilate. There is not enough time in the day for busy practitioners to be cost effective. Some prescribers use drugs that have been found to be less effective than others. Valerian, hops, and chamomile are among the many herbs that are more effective and have little or no side effects.

For those individuals who have not been helped by
traditional medicine, some of these facts may explain the lack of
expected responses and the need to apply Wellness Strategies and
alternatives to integrate a comprehensive approach towards
improvement. Sleep is essential for such pain control and quality
sleep is even more important!

The major non-drug approaches that work best fall into
eight broad categories:

- Wellness Strategies and Natural Energy usage
- Relaxation training
- Cognitive/behavioral techniques
- Biofeedback.
- Nutritionals and Herbs
- Water
- Exercise
- Sleep

One of the more widely used techniques is the application
of natural energy products in conjunction with the use of Wellness
Strategies. This is the Ecology approach to personal health and
pain management. This Ecology Program allows the patient to
have total control over the improvement of their health and the
development of a better quality of life. Using natural energy
products and techniques allows the body to heal and enrich itself
by using the LifeForce Energy that exists in every person and
which is a key component of nature and our environment. Low
dose magnetics, far infrared wraps and comforters, and a pocket
sized, automatic, self-administered electrical nerve and muscle
stimulator alone or in combination are extremely effective for

acute and chronic discomfort. They are worn or taped on the affected areas, sat on as a seat, slept on as a sleep system, or applied directly or indirectly through air or water. Noticeable and significant improvement of symptoms or signs in 50-80% of cases of low back conditions and numbness in the feet and hands is seen, even when those same people are on maximum traditional therapies. In cases of tension and sinus discomfort, relief can be dramatic in up to 100% of cases, however in vascular head discomfort the results are less (50-80%). When Wellness Strategies are used with natural energy, you have the complete ability to change and enrich your personal environment and develop your own Wellness Ecosystem.

The second most popular approach is progressive muscle relaxation. People are taught to slowly tense and relax major muscle groups, typically starting with their feet and progressing up through their trunk, arms, and head. Gradually you can learn to pinpoint signs of tension and get very skilled at just letting it go. It is probably one of the most effective pain control methods we have.

Most cognitive techniques help people divert attention from the pain. Using guided imagery, for example, a therapist will have people imagine themselves in a pleasant scene, telling them: "You can hear the gulls, you can taste the salt on your lips, you can feel the warmth of the sand." You try to get them very involved in the entire experience. Other cognitive strategies challenge how people think about pain. If you are saying things like "I'm worthless," or "There's no hope for me," or "No one really cares", it probably is contributing to your distress and pain. Behavioral techniques are used to alter people's routines. "Activity-rest Cycling," for example, teaches a person to pace their activity. So, rather than attempting to do all their housework in one day, people set up a daily schedule, with periods of activity alternating with rest breaks.

They gradually increase the overall amount they are able to do each day, yet do not experience the peaks of painfulness as they did before.

Biofeedback techniques use monitoring devices to give patients physiological information about their bodies. An electromyograph, for example, can help you recognize and control a muscle spasm that causes recurrent neck pain. If you look at the research, however, it appears that part of the effect is related to the cognitive changes that occur. As you start to control that muscle tension, you begin to believe you can control your body. That sense of mastery explains outcomes better in many cases than the actual physiological changes.

Self-efficacy is very important. It is the belief that you have the capability to engage in behavior that will change your response to pain. You can have self-efficacy by telling yourself you can control severe pain. On the other hand, you might have self-efficacy by insisting, "Even in the face of pain, I can put on my clothes and work a couple of hours". Research suggests that among people having similar degrees of physical damage, those with higher levels of self-efficacy will have a lot less pain.

To get the best results from all of the above systems, it is best to adopt a program that combines a "menu" of options. By developing a personal menu, a LifeForce Wellness Strategy Plan, one can compliment the main system with an interdisciplinary team that may include one or more health care providers and a wellness consultant that integrates the best of eastern and western thinking.

Pain is easily defined; you know it when you feel it. It is that ugly relative who comes to visit and then takes over your life. However, the scientific definition of pain, according to the

35

International Association for the Study of Pain, defines it as "an unpleasant sensory and emotional experience associated with actual or potential tissue damage or described in terms of such damage". The key thing is that pain is both sensory and emotional. It is not just a physical phenomenon.

You can have pain in the absence of physical pathology, which can be true in cases of up to 85 percent of people with back pain and over 20% of those who have seen multiple consultants without a positive response and 95 percent of people who have headaches. Pain is subjective, that each individual interprets it for himself or herself. Pain is always real to the individual, so there is no way you can say it's "psychological" or not real. It is what a person tells you.

We have to make a distinction between simple sensory information, such as the prick of a pin, and the more complex perception of pain that results when sensory information is filtered through an individual's experience, mood, or expectations. Two individuals who experience the same amount of noxious stimulation may interpret it very differently depending on a host of psychological factors.

The most convincing explanation is the "gate control" theory that dates back to the 1960s. "Gate Control" simply advocates that sensory information coming from the body's periphery may be transmitted through the spinal cord to the brain directly. As the result of certain emotions or other cognitive factors, however, the brain may send a signal down the spinal cord that "closes a gate" and prevents that information from ever getting into sensory awareness. People have modified the original theory, but the general conceptual model holds to this day. The anatomy, the physiology, the neurochemistry of pain –" those we're still wrestling with".

The bottom line is that pain is an environmental creature that is easily influenced by a number of ecological factors from the weather to social/emotional interactions. Prior learning experience is a common one. Go out to a playground and watch what happens when a child falls down. It is guaranteed that the closer he gets to mom, the louder the crying, and the more tears you are going to see. In addition, how mom responds is going to have an impact the next time the child has pain. Gender differences are also part of the ecology mix.

Chronic pain patients generally fall into three categories: "Dysfunctional" patients are in severe pain, have a high level of emotional distress, and feel they have little control over their lives. "Interpersonally distressed" patients also have severe pain, but say they get very negative responses from significant people around them. "Adaptive copers" deal much better with their severe pain. They have much less emotional distress and tend to be more active.

Thus, an individual who is dysfunctional might need a treatment that is quite different from someone who has interpersonal problems, which might in turn be very different from the treatment you offer someone who is coping pretty well. However, all three types will significantly benefit from Natural LifeForce Energy usage and the daily use of Wellness Strategies, because of the environmental nature of pain that all three types share in common.

Because the nature of pain is environmental, most people suffer frequently from pain that results from a series of learned behaviors.

There is a definite distinction between "pain" and "pain behavior" - the actions of someone in pain. A person who feels pain, they said, may take medication, receive help from a spouse, or reduce activity with each occurrence. Each positive response tends to reinforce the pain behavior, so that over time the patient may continue to feel pain even after the injury heals.

Extensive research has clearly revealed that natural energy usage and Wellness Strategies (along with relaxation and cognitive-behavioral approaches) is effective in treating tension-type headaches and that the outcomes rival those for drug treatments. Further, the good effects can last several years. In addition, adequate nutrition, herbs, clean filtered water, proper exercise, and quality sleep all affect the body's ability to maintain and restore balance to lessen both physical and mental pain.

Ø Ø Ø

3. Workplace Stress: Your Job May Be Killing You

Job strain that leads to physical illness has become an unpleasant fact for millions of workers worldwide. Almost half of all working Americans report they are highly concerned about job-related stress, and reports from workers in other industrial countries echo this cry, with all too serious health consequences. Scores of studies have shown high stress on the job generates greater risk of coronary heart disease. Immune disorders, back pain, and mental and emotional strain are other clearly demonstrated risks. Individuals must and should take steps to reduce and cope with the stress in their lives, and incorporating LifeForce usage and Wellness Strategies is the only pro-active solution both at work and at home.

The Facts‡:

- Workers in jobs that give them little latitude in decision-making had a 50 percent higher rate of coronary heart disease than those with high job control.

- Also, there is a more than twofold risk for new coronary heart disease among people who make a high level of personal effort on the job but receive little in the way of recognition or promotions.

- Unemployment creates health risks. Even a serious threat of unemployment triggers physiological effects linked to heart disease. Evidence from several countries demonstrates those unemployed persons and their families run a substantially increased risk of premature death.

- Women tend to experience job strain differently from men, for many reasons. One is that many of their jobs involve actions that must be repeated precisely every few seconds, as in cookie factories and clothing manufacturers.

- Many Americans have been blinded by the media myth that associates job stress with Type A behavior. Others, however, believe that workloads and environmental demands led to high stress.

However, the problem has two dimensions. One relates to the demands of the work, particularly the mental and psychological demands. The other measures the control the individual has over the demands in that situation. These factors lead to two other components: (1) bad stress and (2) good stress. When the demands are high and the individual has little control over them, the negative consequences of strain or stress develop. There is increased risk of physical illness and diverse negative emotional states. This is "Bad Stress"!

Good stress results from the following: as long as the job demands are not too overwhelmingly high and there are high levels of individual job control, there usually are feelings of satisfaction, motivation, and possibilities of learning new things - that is, challenging work - even new coping strategies that could prevent illness.

Social support is a major factor that forms a third independent dimension. So now the effects of "good stress" and "bad stress" are measured by analyzing the factors of psychological and physical demands of the job, the individual's decisional latitude, the level of job insecurity, and social support.

Many studies have shown significant ties to absenteeism, mental disorders, immune system disorders, and musculoskeletal problems, such as repetitive strain injuries, which usually do not have only physical causes. Psychosocial factors also play a large role.

Certainly, there are individually based solutions that provide short-term stress relief, but we need to begin thinking about long-term, social solutions. We are seeing huge amounts of mental strain, heart disease, immune system disorders, musculoskeletal disorders, absenteeism, and other problems. They involve enormous human suffering and huge costs to modern society. These are vital social/political issues, and they should be part of our political discussion of how our society and the economy should work. However, they are not, certainly not in the United States. America has turned into the Blind, Deaf, and Dumb Monkeys when it comes to the importance of wellness to the security of our country and society.

There are ways to improve workers' control over their situations, their pace of work, their tools, and the methods they use in the workplace. For one thing, it is important to have open communication. This requires an organizational culture that fosters trust, and of course trust does not come from slogans - it comes from demonstrated behaviors at the company.

Incentives of various kinds could be given to companies to set up programs for work groups to discuss their sources of stress in the workplace and how to consider them. The "health circles" in some German workplaces do this very effectively. We should try them here. We have been willing to adopt management strategies

41

that increase job stress from any country in the world, but when it comes time to protect ourselves from job stress we say, "No, that can't work here".

Employees also need to feel that social and political processes in which they are shareholders in the company can influence the company, not just by decisions of financial powers that may decide to close down the factory tomorrow.

What is needed is, first, good collaboration among co-workers and a feeling of trust with curbs on harassment of different types. Secondly, a value system that goes beyond dollars and cents, e.g., doctors and nurses who are trained to take good care of patients, not just cut costs.

Improved health is consistent with improving productivity, but only of a certain kind - productivity associated with increased human capabilities, increased skill, increasing effective collaboration. These are indeed the productivity areas of the future. Witness, the Internet; innovative product development; networked production; education; and health care in its true forms. Thus, there are large-scale social solutions to stress problems that could work.

A work environment can be designed that is low in job stress! None of us yet knows exactly what makes a work environment ideal, safe, and healthful, but many of us are trying to put a name to it, so we can begin to explore it. What is clear is that the focus should be at the level of the organization, because you are trying to understand something that is bigger than any one individual.

It is a lot like a related area of research that has had more attention - neighborhoods that are supportive or detrimental to health. You usually start by taking a sample of people in the neighborhood, asking them about how supportive and trusting their neighbors are. "Would your neighbor help you out in a fix?" "Would you trust your neighbor to call you if your kid wasn't in school one day?" Moreover, you go on from there.

That could be one starting point, but there are others. For example "surrogate" approaches, such as looking at job appraisals rather than the environment itself. This comes from the idea that their supervisors in work environments will rate employees favorably where people have a high level of perceived control over their jobs and an appropriate level of work demand. In work environments that are very autocratic, you are likely to see many unfavorable ratings.

Of course, we also look into the environment itself to see what may be either a protective factor or an accelerator of bad stress. We have some strong presentiments about what it is about a work environment that might be good for your health, but from a scientific point of view, it is all still quite untested.

This has something to do with the whole relationship that exists between employees and their work environment. Some of the environments are life support structures for the people lucky enough to be working in them. They have absolutely low rates of serious chronic diseases. In some facilities the risk of disease appears to be no better than in the population as a whole, and perhaps even worse.

The challenge is to figure out what it is we can change. We cannot triple the workers' income or quickly modify all their good or bad habits or change their diets. However, we can educate them and make the work environment different, and that is part of the thrust of this whole research line.

The idea is not new. What is new is the way we are going to do it. First we will try to do the science. If the science works, we will try to do the interventions to make things better.

Women are more likely than men to bring job stress home. Scientific studies are starting to figure out why. These studies show that some women's jobs often involve a large number of what may look like insignificant difficulties but add up to a high level of job stress, higher than that associated with men's jobs. Women's higher job stress at home may be a combination of less job control and more at-home responsibilities. Which means women are thinking more about their life at home while they are on the job and more conscious of their jobs when they are at home.

Building those bridges is the number one problem reported by workingwomen who have children, and it is getting close to the top for men, too. It is not just that women have more responsibility for childcare and housekeeping. Women's jobs are also more likely to be rigidly structured; so many of them cannot take the time to make a doctor's appointment or find a sitter when childcare arrangements falter.

Society does not judge women entirely on what they do at work, whereas men's traditional sense of self is based on conducting their work life well and being a good provider. Thus, women generally do not feel the terrible pressure that men feel to ensure economic survival with their jobs. Not many women commit suicide because they have been fired or go around shooting everybody up.

More than 54 percent of American workers are either "very" or "extremely" concerned about stress from work demands, and 88 percent of them say the amount of stress they feel on the job is an important factor.

The ability to balance work and family is the number one priority cited by those surveyed – more important than job security, quality of working environment, and relationships with co-workers and supervisors.

Eighty-seven percent of the workers reported they are concerned with getting enough sleep, with 60 percent saying they are very or extremely concerned about it.

Ø Ø Ø

4. Sleep

Quality sleep is truly the foundation of great health. Every day we put physical stress on our muscles, joints, and internal systems. In addition, the mind gets a workout as well. Sleep is the body's way of restoring itself, to get ready for the next day. Miss the sleep you need and you are taxing your body's defenses. Lack of sleep has been implicated as a major contributor to illness. In addition, many medical specialists consider it a major health problem today. According to a 1999 survey conducted by the National Sleep Foundation, nearly half of us have trouble sleeping several times a week—difficulty in falling asleep, waking up too many times or feeling tired in the morning. Over 30% of people have chronic problems sleeping. Moreover, almost all of us have these problems from time to time. Years of research and testing have identified the exact requirements for a person to sleep well. Nikken, an international wellness company, has incorporated these findings into their advanced technology sleep system. The components are an orthopedically designed contoured pillow; a mattress pad or mattress that contains specially designed magnets, memory foam, proprietary rubberthane on an egg crate type surface, and a far-infrared comforter with bioceramic fibers.

The new Dream Sleep System ™ also incorporates negative ion generation technology for health promotion and chitosan into the fibers of the comforter, providing properties that adversely affect pathogenic organisms and favor allergic prone individuals. This system delivers a sleep that you will look forward to for the rest of your life. The main benefit is an increase of quality sleep. Many people feel completely rested and can have one hour less of sleep every night and not miss it—a dramatic productivity boost over a working lifetime. How would you like to have over 300 extra hours per year to play or work?

People who rely on powers of concentration such as chess players and research scientists will typically notice a significant improvement in their level of performance and endurance. The same is true for endeavors where physical stamina is required such as professional sports where an extra edge and rapid recovery time is important.

Children also can benefit from more daily energy and better sleep quality, especially those with attention and focus challenges as well as autistic behaviors. Improved academic performance may become dramatic and behavior with less stress may result.

UNFORTUNATELY THOSE WITH PACEMAKERS OR OTHER IMPLANTED DEVICES CAN NOT SLEEP ON MAGNETIC PADS OF ANY KIND SINCE THE DEVICE COULD BE TRIGGERED OFF. Women in the first trimester (first 3 months) should not use magnets and should check with their physician for other times. Even though there never has been a documented history of any serious consequences in pregnancy, manufacturers and health care providers should always be consulted.

It is a prudent decision to invest in an essential health product on which you spend 1/3 of your life. This is much safer than taking sleeping pills that can cause numerous side effects and are not good for you. Milk or an aspirin before bedtime may help some people. Herbals such as valerian, hops, and chamomile may also help. More progressive and innovative use of natural energy incorporates magnetics, far-infrared, negative ion generation, and chitosan cotton to provide the ultimate in comfort, safety, and efficacy for restful and quality sleep with recuperative enhancement of the mind and body. This is the way to go.

5. Mind/Body Behavior

Heart disease is the number one killer of both adult men and women in the United States and the leading cause of permanent disability from the work force. Certain aspects of behavior -- including diet, smoking, and a sedentary lifestyle -- increase the chances that heart disease will develop or get worse. Various psychological factors -- such as hostility, anger, stress, and depression -- also increase risk. A number of cognitive and behavioral strategies have been used successfully to keep people on their diet and exercise regimes and to teach them ways to counter the effects of stress and a coronary-prone personality. When these strategies are employed in a comprehensive program that targets multiple risk factors, people stand the best chance of avoiding a heart attack or preventing another cardiac event.

The Facts‡:

- Heart disease afflicts more than 12.2 million people in the United States and is the single largest cause of death among both men and women and the leading cause of premature, permanent disability.

- Heart disease costs the U.S. economy $214.7 billion a year, including $105.9 billion in direct treatment costs and $108.8 billion in lost productivity due to illness or death.

- A number of psychological factors significantly increase the risk of developing heart disease or help speed its progression, including stress, Type A behavior, hostility, depression, and social isolation. Stress management skills, relaxation techniques, and other behavioral treatments can reduce the risk

49

of death from heart disease among those at risk of developing heart disease as well as those with established illness.

- Although women frequently express greater fear of breast cancer than heart disease, more than eight times as many women die each year from heart disease, making it the number one cause of death among women. Women who have had heart attacks are significantly less likely than men to undergo invasive diagnostic procedures, such as cardiac catheterization, or to receive clot-busting drugs, angioplasty, or bypass surgery to improve blood flow to their hearts.

- Women take significantly longer to seek care for heart attack symptoms than do men -- 6.2 hours for women vs. 5.4 hours for men, in one recent study. Differences in the symptoms that women experience compared with men may explain the added delay. Women are significantly more likely than men to describe their chest pain as "pressure," "heaviness," or "tightness," but are significantly less likely than men to report the more "classic" pain in the center or left side of their chest. Women are also more likely to report other symptoms not related to chest pain, including back pain, nausea, vomiting, indigestion, and shortness of breath.

- Patients with heart disease who completed an intensive lifestyle modification program were able to reduce significantly the narrowing in their coronary arteries without taking cholesterol-lowering medications.

Heart disease affects tens of millions of Americans in one-way or another. There are 10 to 12 million people with angina (chest pain that occurs when the heart muscle does not receive enough blood). There are a 1.5 million heart attacks each year and in excess of 750,000 coronary revascularization procedures, such as bypass surgery and angioplasty. As the population ages, heart

50

disease stands to become an even larger problem. African Americans and Native Americans are more likely than other groups to suffer from hypertension and diabetes -- two conditions that increase the risk for heart disease. Contrary to popular belief, women have about the same rate of death from coronary artery disease as men do. Women acquire the disease somewhat later in life, but they also tend to live longer than men do. However, heart disease is very preventable.

There are three components to basic Wellness: education, group support, and skills training. First, teach people about risk factors and the role of stress and its effects on the body. The second component is social support. Stress management training is done in groups where people can share their frustrations and their successes and see they are not alone in facing these challenges. The third component includes a variety of different skills to cope with stress, ranging from relaxation training to teaching people different cognitive behavioral strategies to help them respond differently to situations that previously were regarded as very stressful. Cognitive behavioral strategies refer to techniques for modifying the ways in which individuals perceive and interpret various situations. People learn to monitor their thought patterns, to recognize when their thinking is not realistic, and to challenge their unrealistic thought patterns and substitute them with more appropriate, realistic, and adaptive cognitions.

The most dangerous risk factor is the Type A personality. People who have Type A personalities tend to be impatient and irritable. They also feel a real sense of time urgency, and they get easily angered. Numerous studies have shown that people with Type A behavior and high levels of hostility show greater heart rate and blood pressure changes and a greater release of certain stress hormones in response to stress.

Ø Ø Ø

51

6. Exercising Your Options: The Benefits Of Physical Activity

Regular physical activity promotes overall health and well-being and can help prevent and treat heart disease and other chronic conditions. Yet despite these proven benefits, two-thirds of Americans do not engage in regular exercise and one-quarter are sedentary. Behavioral interventions can help people become and remain active. Among the strategies that can help individuals adopt and continue an active lifestyle are brief counseling sessions with a physician, educational materials tailored to people's individual motivation to change, and the creation of safe and convenient venues where people can be active.

The Facts‡:

• Two-thirds of American adults do not achieve recommended levels of physical activity in their daily lives. Those recommendations urge all adults to accumulate 30 minutes or more of moderate-intensity physical activity on most, and preferably all, days of the week or 20 or more minutes of vigorous-intensity activity at least three days a week.

• Regular physical activity reduces the risk of developing high blood pressure, heart disease, diabetes, and colon cancer. It also helps control weight, reduces feelings of depression and anxiety, and can help older adults avoid falls by remaining stronger and more mobile.

• About one-quarter of American adults do not engage in any leisure-time physical activity.

- Nearly half of all young people age 12 to 21 are not vigorously active on a regular basis, and 14 percent report no recent physical activity.

- Job-site health promotion programs show promise in improving levels of physical activity among workers.

- Many patients increase their activity after brief counseling by their physician.

Physical activity is so important because, in addition to the previously known role of exercise in reducing the risk of obesity, hypertension, heart disease, stroke, and diabetes, newer studies suggest it also may be linked with reductions in breast, colon, and other cancers. We also know that physical activity can be a health and performance enhancing behavior, improving your mood and how you feel about yourself, as well as how you perform at work or interact with your family. Therefore, the importance is not only in preventing disease, but also in optimizing health and functional capability for people.

Physical inactivity is a big problem, reaching epidemic proportions because over two-thirds of the population is not doing enough exercise or physical activity. Guidelines from the Centers for Disease Control and Prevention (CDC) and the American College of Sports Medicine (ACSM) were originally designed to help people reach a particular level of cardiovascular fitness. They recommend that people accumulate at least 30 minutes of moderate physical activity a day on five or more days a week. The guidelines expand physical activity beyond the realm of exercise and account for all the activities a person might do during the day. Your 30 minutes of activity a day might include 10 minutes walking up and down stairs to and from your office, a 10-minute walk at lunch, and 10 minutes raking leaves when you get home.

It is really is quite easy for anyone to undertake a home-based exercise program. In fact, patients who exercised at home spent more time on their exercise bicycles than patients who were randomized to the gym program spending time in their car and driving to and from the gym. Many people do not have access to gyms or do not like group exercise programs. For them, exercise training at home is a very attractive alternative. An easy walking program on a daily basis is provided with a properly constructed weighted sole in a tennis type walking shoe that assists in back, hip, knee, ankle, and foot alignment and is currently only made by Nikken. They are called CardioStrides™ and increase metabolism and can assist in weight reduction. Inactive people who do not like to exercise will love them.

Recent guidelines are more focused on behavior -- getting people off the couch and starting to do something. The evidence is very clear that there is a health benefit to physical activity that does not meet the cardiovascular fitness guidelines. Therefore, when someone goes from being pretty sedentary to active, the decrease in disease risk is dramatic. They may still benefit from more vigorous activity, but the greatest benefit comes from simply becoming physically active.

Most people have difficulty remaining physically active because many people say they have a lack of time or are not able to build it into their daily routine. Others say it is too expensive to join a health club or purchase home exercise equipment. In the end, a lot of these barriers can be overcome with adequate support from friends or family members. If you are not anxious to exercise, you can walk with the weighted CardioStrides™ shoes starting out walking for 10 minutes and gradually increasing the time daily until you are walking in them all day and burning calories effortlessly.

Ø Ø Ø

7. Good Nutrition

Diet is a key determinant of health and an important contributor to chronic disease and premature death. Although progress has been made in improving the U.S. population's diet during the past few decades, a large gap between consumers' eating practices and public health recommendations persists. Individualized behavioral and educational approaches, such as counseling and computer-tailored messages, may help some people to improve their diets. Many experts assert, however, that social, policy and professional education changes are needed as well.

The Facts‡:

• Diet is an important, controllable risk factor for five leading causes of death: heart disease, some types of cancer, stroke, diabetes, and coronary artery disease. Diet also plays a role in a person's risk of hypertension, high blood cholesterol, osteoporosis and gallbladder disease.

• Experts estimate that unhealthful eating and physical inactivity are responsible for more than 300,000 premature deaths each year in the United States.

• Today, 55 percent of U.S. adults 20 or older are overweight or obese. Ten percent to 15 percent of young people 6 to 17 years old are overweight.

• Obesity in the U.S. population increased from 12 percent in 1991 to 18 percent in 1998.

57

- While the average daily intake of fruits and vegetables consumed by Americans has risen, only 35 percent of the population meets the goal of eating five servings of fruits and vegetable a day.

- Intake of total fat, saturated fat, cholesterol, and sodium remains above recommended levels, while calcium intake and iron intake remain below recommended levels for many population groups.

- Poor nutrition and malnutrition are by-products of our cultural obsession with beauty.

The American Heart Association guidelines recommend eating more plant-based foods rather than counting calories and adding two servings a week of fish--particularly those high in omega-3 fatty acids, notably salmon and tuna--to a diet already rich in fruits, vegetables, legumes, whole grains, low-fat dairy products, fish, lean meats and poultry.

Soy, Supplements, And Herbs - With a balanced diet, nutritional supplementation, and herbs to enhance well-being and optimum health, providing the body with high-octane fuel increases the prevention of disease and aging. In addition, the body is better able to heal itself naturally when trauma, cancer, and other diseases attack it.

It has been noted that a diet rich in soy protein appears to decrease inflammation induced pain. It can also be preventative for many cancers. Two-thirds of patients with advanced cancer suffer from chronic pain due to tissue infiltration and inflammation and neuropathic pain from tumors invading a nerve bed.   Cancer cells can also release chemicals that trigger painful responses. It also has been noted that cancer cells are adversely affected by an alkaline and oxygen enriched environment so that water that is slightly alkaline and superoxygenated would theoretically be preventative. Studies at Hopkins are currently being conducted to validate earlier studies on dietary soy for pain control.

Because of soil depletion despite crop rotation, many fruits and vegetables are depleted of nutrients necessary for optimum health so supplementation is necessary, especially when most of the population does not eat healthy foods properly.

Companies are few which provide the necessary vitamins and minerals in the correct proportions along with antioxidants that are personalized or mixed and matched for different ages or conditions and are of pharmaceutical grade, bioavailable, and absorbable. If they are synergistic and biodirected with natural energy products that have magnetic and/or far infrared features, it is another advantage!

Herbs are generally safe and do not need monitoring. They may be adaptogens, which enhance multiple body systems. In many cases they can be used in place of pharmaceuticals. They are usually indigenous to locations where the local people have to be consulted in their application since they have worked very well for them and their ancestors for thousands of years without any scientific studies. Changing one's diet is the least risky method of managing a lot of chronic diseases and related risk factors like hypertension and high blood cholesterol. It also is a lot less expensive than most pharmacologic types of treatment. For instance, a person who has high blood pressure and is overweight and not eating a healthy diet often can bring his or her blood pressure under control through dietary changes, without taking medicine. On the other hand, if a person is on medication, a healthier diet may reduce the amount of medication needed and in some cases eliminate the need for pharmaceuticals

Nutrition has many qualitative dimensions. You need to look at whether people are eating fruits and vegetables, how high their fat intake is, whether they are eating too many calories or whether they are getting enough calcium. The measures that are easiest to report on are weight and obesity. In the United States, about half the adults are either overweight or obese.

More healthful foods, such as fat-modified foods, are available than in the past, but there also is a trend toward eating more rich, high-calorie, high-sugar, high-fat foods. One important dimension of the problem in the United States is that portion sizes are becoming larger. For example, a bagel nowadays is about twice the size of what it was 10 or 15 years ago.

It is typically thought that if we can get people to eat more fruits and vegetables, people will not eat as much of the unhealthy foods. People coming from different disease perspectives generally agree upon that approach. The other approach is to reduce the overall quantity of food individuals consume to bring it closer to the amount of energy they expend.

Across the board, taste came out at the top. Cost was the second most important influence. Certain clusters of people said nutrition and weight control were more important, but overall, taste was ranked the most important. Part of the take-home message from this finding is that if people want to eat tasty foods and we want them to eat healthy foods, then we have to find ways to make nutritious foods tastier.

Here are some of the barriers to nutritious eating: Limitations on people's time is certainly one. Access to and availability of healthful food choices is another barrier for some people -- if they are on the road, at work or in a part of the country where fresh foods are not available.

As a society, we tend to be much more rushed with less time for food preparation, and there are more options for take-away foods. These foods are often higher in fat, salt, and calories than the homemade equivalents. Although they need not be less healthy, they often are.

People who have a real driving reason to change are most successful; for instance, if they have just been diagnosed with high cholesterol. In this situation, a message from a doctor, such as, "If your blood pressure doesn't go down, we'll put you on medication," or "You're diabetic and you're going to lose your eyesight if we don't get this under control," can be very motivating.

Sometimes people are motivated by other factors, such as friends' health problems, not feeling well and the positive feelings they might get by improving their diet for a little while. It is not easy to suggest one motivator for all people, but these are some examples that "hit the mark" for some.

People have generally gotten the message about eating fewer fats, more fruits, and vegetables and less salt. The much more difficult piece for people is knowing how to apply the knowledge -- knowing what to buy, how to read the labels and how to put together a meal that reflects the recommendations. Even harder is getting people to make changes and stick with them on a long-term basis. People need to understand that there is no magic bullet approach of one food or one change that will extend their lives.

Ø Ø Ø

8. Water

William Nusz *(Trainer for the U.S. Koshiki Karate Team)*
My Experiences with the Benefits of Natural Energy:

It has been said that water is the source of inspiration for the method of winning. Water is shapeless and conforming yet has the force to erode stone or crush an object. It also helps to sustain life!

Karate is an art. Karatedo is a way of life, my way of life or "LifeForce" since 1967 when I started my Martial Arts training. For my martial arts training, I owe my deepest gratitude to my Sensei (teacher), Kaicho, Shunji Watanabe, and my head master, Hanshi (professor), So Shihan Masayuki Kukan Hisataka, heir to the Shorinjiryu Kenkokan style and the founder of the Koshiki Karatedo system. Through them, I was also taught what I consider to be the art of living. That is, how to overcome situations of conflict in daily life with the underlying principles of many classic martial traditions such as, the Gokyo or Five Teachings: Water, (Mizu); Fire, (Hi); Earth, (Chi); Wind, (Kaze); and Air or Emptiness, (Ku). These teachings are timeless.

During the late 1500's and early 1600's in Japanese history, Miyamoto Musashi, the most famous Samurai (protector of the clan) of the time, wrote about these principles in his book "Gorin No Sho" ("the Book of Five Rings"), including a section on Water as it related to the use of the sword. The sword was also called the soul of the Samurai. Being fluid in movement and

63

flexible, with the ability to adapt or conform to its surroundings, this is "Mizu"(water) which goes with the flow.

In my style of the martial arts, Shorinjiryu Kenkokan Karate, the first teaching, Dia Ikkyo, stresses the mental state of mizu no kokoro, mind of water. The mind of water, to be calm, is for me the most important state of mind one can achieve at home, at work or in the dojo (training hall). It has helped me in times of stress and discomfort. Along with that, water is my source of energy, and how the body cleanses itself. I have with me at all times, a self filtering water bottle, a combination of ionic filtration, pi ceramics, and magnetic and far-infrared technologies, that take out the impurities and gives me the proper elements of water needed to live well, work and train harder. When I travel, in the United States or throughout the world, the bottle goes with me, ensuring me good clean, healthy water. Why take chances!

In 1996, I trained a team and traveled to Japan to represent the United States in the 15th Japan Open Koshiki Karate Championship. This was my last tournament as a participant. I finished 3rd for a bronze medal in the Men's Black Belt Kata (forms) division but did not do as well in the Shiai (sparring) division. I broke my wrist and tore ligaments that I found out later were beyond repair. Mizu No Kokoro, be calm, forget the pain and go with the flow all came to mind. When I returned to the States I underwent three surgeries on my wrist and received a new cast every month for 14 months. The last three months I wore an electro-magnetic bone stimulator on the cast 10 hours a day for bone growth and it worked! The wrist mended but now I only have limited flexibility of my right wrist that I will have to deal with the rest of my life. When the last cast came off I was in agony, the kind that keeps you awake at night. I was then introduced to Dr. Lee Gresser, who took the discomfort away without medication within two hours. He put two tiny magnetic discs on my wrist, one on the top and one on the bottom, and wrapped the wrist with a support wrap designed with far-infrared technology, to control the healing area temperature. I have been using these products ever since. Dr.Gresser introduced magnetic health, far-infrared technologies and products to my students and now is our team doctor.

Since the tournament in Japan, I have traveled as an International Referee to Canada, Switzerland and Australia using several magnetic products and of course my water bottle. Dr. Gresser traveled with the team to Australia and used natural energy magnetic products to enhance the mobility, range of motion, speed and strength of the competitors as well as to speed up the recovery rate of those who were injured. This not only impressed the attending tournament staff medics, it was of great help to them during the event. Since then, newer products and technologies have been released, enhancing the performance of many students in the martial arts. The next tournament will be in Lisbon, Portugal, November 2003, where we will again be using products of natural energy.

Shihan William Nusz, *Renshi* (6th degree black belt)
International Referee, Trainer, US Koshiki Karatedo Team
President, US Shorinjiryu Kenkokan Karatedo / US Koshiki Karatedo Federations
President, Nihon Takaiyama Karatedo, Inc.

http://www.geocities.com/nihon_takaiyama/
shihannusz@yahoo.com

The Importance of "Better" Water: With over
70% of the body being water, the purity of the water and its natural energy is essential for life. Adequate hydration is necessary for movement of blood cells, oxygen, nutrition, the body's immune defense system, vitamins, minerals enzymes, etc. towards every cell and organ system. With dehydration the restorative process is hampered and disease can take over. If we had water from high in the Andes mountains where there was no significant acid rain, soil runoff and contamination, and pathogens from air, soil, and animals, we would have the optimum water that becomes magnetized naturally by running down brooks and streams and is filtered by natural stones and ceramics in river beds. We have been able to produce such water through advanced technological processes, including a unique filtering and treatment system through Nikken. This water is called Pi-Mag™ water and is available in a sports or flip-top bottle (refillable) with its own self-contained filtering system and magnetic and far infrared tote. It is also available in a counter top unit that attaches to your faucet (delivers at least 1200 gallons of drinking water and requires a change of filters every 1-2 years depending on usage and number of people in the household). A unique recent addition of a gravity fed portable "dripolator" type unit holds 2.6 gallons of water without plumbing or electric. It allows in a short period of time the production of similar clean, filtered, treated, energized water which can be obtained at half the cost of the sink unit. It can then be superoxygenated, alkalinized, and magnetically enhanced to increase easier transport of nutritionals into cells by a device called the "Optimizer" which looks and acts like a blender with magnets. Because magnetic energy affects every living cell in people, pets, and plants and ions have to move in a liquid medium, the main deterrent for a clinically positive response is dehydration. So Drink Plenty of Good Clean Water!

9. *Wellness and Martial Arts: Training For Health & Life*

The Japanese had an interest in the training of the warrior class and approached the problem in an empirical and practical way, basing their psychology on observable behavior and concrete achievements in contest and battle. The training goals of the martial arts are slightly different from what most people expect from sports. The aim of training is never mere technical excellence or efficiency. That is merely a byproduct of the development of perfect form and concentration. The discipline of the martial arts was so demanding that it reshaped the student mentally and physically in every action. A man or woman who achieved mastery of an art would show this in their every action. The idea was to develop concentration and attention and to control the emotions, especially fear and anxiety.

The method of training involved little stress on intellectual explanation. Direct experience was most important. Teachers showed students the value of self-control directly. They did not just talk about it. Mental development was highly valued, especially over mere technical skill. The teachers deliberately set out to improve physical skills through mental discipline by developing the powers of attention and concentration, and by eliminating the fear and nervousness that will inhibit performance. Fear and anxiety, in small amounts may increase performance, but in larger doses will make it much more difficult to distinguish danger from trivia. Fear also causes greater rigidity in the response pattern that becomes more stereotyped and habitual. Reducing fear involves eliminating the fear of dying, and making a calm mind by creating a balanced and relaxed body. Learning to work with the

67

hara, the lower abdomen, which is also the physical center of balance, is critical to this.

Mental health is not just the absence of illness, but is an overall sense of wellness, in body and mind. Much of the recent self-help and human growth interest concentrates on Eastern approaches that recognize this idea. The underlying reality of Martial arts is explained as self- discipline, self-awareness, control, mind-body harmony, mental strength, relaxation, and personal development. The training is designed to improve mental discipline, concentration, relaxation, self-awareness, and the feeling of personal competence. It is not mainly about physical skills. There are several ways of looking at martial arts: as an art form giving grace and inner expression, as meditation, as a competitive contact or non-contact sport, or as kickboxing. Traditional training focuses on the art/meditative aspects while "modern" training concentrates on the sport/competitive aspect. Traditional training gives little time to tournament competition stressing mainly mental discipline, character, and physical skills. The motto of the Shorinjiryu Kenkokan Karate schools is "Spiritual Development of Individuality in Mind and Body", stressing that the mind and body must act as one.

It should be of great interest to those dealing with gender issues that martial arts training create an equality between the sexes, at least with regard to gender identification within each person. It has often been suggested that a more feminine male would be more sensitive to women's issues and it would perhaps be reasonable to assume that a more masculine woman would be more understanding of men.

Any period of martial arts training is enough to raise self-esteem. The self-perception of ability relates to self-esteem. Self-perception of physical condition and self- discipline was also

68

important to self-esteem, and self-esteem predicted performance. Martial arts students have a realistic appreciation of their own abilities, and that possession of these abilities is related to their self-esteem. Training in martial arts does not result in unrealistic appraisals of one's abilities.

Those who are less extraverted, who are more susceptible to conditioning and are inclined to live their lives within relatively precise and narrow parameters are predisposed to reach the higher grades of martial arts which is a highly ordered and personal art form.

Wellness Therapy And Martial Arts: One of the most often stated goals of training in the martial arts is to reduce aggression and increase self-control. In older studies, two opposing theories on aggression were often proposed. The catharsis theory attempted to explain a reduction in aggression through combat arts by supposing that these arts provided a socially acceptable way to act out violence, thus "bleeding off" the impulses. The circular theory assumed that aggression is increased through exposure to aggression. The position of these two theories in sociological research has been discussed.

The anthropological lesson from non-literate societies is clear. Whatever genetic potential we may have for aggressive behavior, early conditioning in cooperative behavior, and the discouragement of anything resembling aggressive behavior serve to make an individual and a society essentially unaggressive and cooperative. It remains to be seen what effect the fighting arts may have on adults, who have gone through their early conditioning, and on children who are still being socialized.

69

The study of martial arts provides an alternative to being either an aggressor or a victim, since the learning of self-defense skills, at least in a traditional martial arts class, does not seem to make one more aggressive. This finding was contrary to the expected finding and supported conventional wisdom. Traditional martial arts training stresses self-control, conflict avoidance, and care for contact allowed during training. Other things which are stressed include kata (patterned movements), meditation, philosophy, and respect for others. Another possible mechanism by which higher belt ranks might become associated with lower aggression is that the instructors slowly ease out aggressive students, thus selecting for low aggression. Dropouts of a traditional school are more aggressive than those who stay. This would suggest a method by which the higher belt levels test less aggressive.

As experience level in the martial arts increases, students show lower anxiety, a higher sense of responsibility, and a decrease in willingness to take risks. They are less "radical", have increased self-esteem, and are more socially intelligent. These trends are especially pronounced in the black belt levels. Other effects are seen in increased physical fitness, defense skills, self-discipline, concentration, and respect. Karate begins and ends with respect.

The martial arts training center is associated with mu, emptiness; "mu is an ego-less state of mind that frees one from fear and failure, even in death." To achieve this state, training in Zen meditation during a martial arts class has tremendous importance. In this respect, a martial arts class can be an "intermediary" between the self, nature, and natural energy.

There are several reasons why the martial arts are becoming more popular.

The first is the influence of movies and magazines, which present a distorted view of the arts. The second is that they satisfy a need. In the liberal arts curriculum there should be the ideal of building the body and mind in harmony. This should be the goal of physical education in any school, not "the big game". Western sports ideals are not appealing to many. The aggressiveness and team spirit may seem wrong. The martial arts training center offers an alternative, providing self-knowledge, self-control, and unity with nature rather than self-satisfaction, the defeat of others, and the control of nature.

Other than teaching self-defense the martial arts training center offers access to Eastern thought and philosophy unencumbered by language and culture. It teaches the five "S":

1. *Self-Discipline*
2. *Self-Training*
3. *Self-Control*
4. *Self-Confidence*
5. *Self-Respect*

The most important aspect of martial arts is mental training to allow a calm response to all situations. A group of stable people can provide great assistance to unstable societies. Some of the other social benefits include the possibility of coeducational practice, rather than segregated sports classes, improvements in aesthetics, posture, dance, and the possibility of almost unlimited self-expression. Finally, it is the aim of all karate students, that your training in karatedo (do meaning "way") should be experienced as a way of life created by you, and for you to search and create something fresh and new, to strive to reach a state of harmony with your environment. Let me share with you the principles of our school, our dojo kun:

71

1. Maintain propriety, etiquette, dignity and grace.
2. Gain self-understanding by tasting the true meaning of combat.
3. Search for pure principles of being, truth, justice and beauty.
4. Exercise positive personality, confidence, courage and determination.
5. Always seek to develop the character further, aiming toward perfection and complete harmony with creation.

These are essential for your "do", your "way" of life.

The Mind Can Help the Body to Heal:

Suppose that you are in a new city and you need to get downtown. Would you sit in your car, call a tow truck to get the car towed downtown or would you fill up the tank (so you have enough gasoline), get directions for downtown from a knowledgeable person, and drive yourself there? If you are reading this, you would say, "What a silly question. Of course, I would drive there. Why would I get myself towed by a tow-truck?"

Similarly, taking a totally passive and dependent approach when it comes to our own treatment should sound silly too. A majority of us think that when we get sick, our sole responsibility consists of making an appointment with a doctor and then the doctor should "tow" us to the destination of recovery. We see our participation limited to taking the magical pill or whatever medical procedure the doctor performs.

To continue with the analogy of a car, while there are car troubles that only a mechanic can fix, once a mechanic fixes it, we have to take the responsibility for its maintenance. If we handle it roughly, or if we do not do a good job of keeping check on the fluids, pressures, get regular tune-ups, etc., we have to bring the car to the service station repeatedly. Just as after the mechanic completes the repairs, we are responsible for car maintenance, so are we for the maintenance of our body after the surgical and/or medical procedures. Following the first few years of our life, nothing is maintenance free in this body.

What about the situations that arise when we have to take the initiative and leadership in correction of a problem? For instance, when the battery is down and booster cables are inoperative, you ask someone to push the car to crank the engine. You ask someone to give you a push, you get in the drivers seat, guide the steering wheel so the vehicle stays on a straight path, and just when the engine begins to crank, you push the gas pedal to get the car rolling on its way. In this scenario, the only role of the other person is to give you a little push, but you are the one who is "in the driver's seat," fully in-charge, monitoring the whole operation.

Similarly, in matters requiring a physician's care, such as high cholesterol, high triglycerides, high blood pressure, the doctor and the medication are there to just give us that little push, but we need to fully participate, involve ourselves actively in all aspects of the treatment, and really take charge of the entire recovery process.

Mind/body medicine, which in recent years is making great strides, informs us about how we can help in our own treatment. Popular publications such as Time magazine recently reported (January 20,2003) what the health community has come to learn— that hormone levels, neurotransmitters and other substances through relaxation, meditation, visualization of being healthy and recovered and other techniques, can have a significant effect on cholesterol, the heart, and chronic discomfort, even if there is no known medical cause of your problem. In other words, you can do a whole lot, especially if your condition is stress- related.

In fact, what we do for prevention or for recovery from illnesses is more important today than it has ever been in the past. In the past, illnesses for the most part were caused by infections. These infections, such as the plague, polio, cholera, smallpox, tuberculosis, pneumonia, etc., were the scourge of humanity. Human beings lived in terror of these illnesses, but there was precious little they could do to protect themselves or recover from these infections.

We are fortunate to live in these times in which medicine has achieved enormous success in controlling infectious diseases. Now the illnesses that afflict us are products of our lifestyle and our every-day behavior. Ironically, the grand success of medical science against infections has left us with the residue of illnesses over which medicine has less control.

For example, we have the most sophisticated techniques available for by-pass surgery in case of a heart problem. However, such a bypass surgery will "bypass' the real problem if the patient doesn't change his or her lifestyle. Soon he or she may require another bypass surgery.

Other examples of lifestyles and behaviors that cause disorders and obstruct recovery concern patients who drink excessively, eat unwisely, do little exercise, let the stress go out of control, and constantly live under negative emotions, such as, hostility, depression, frustration, etc. Avoid health-risk behaviors. Practice good-health behaviors, such as relaxation, health-visualization, exercise, wise eating, positive emotions, playing, and laughing.

Mind/body medicine is not a substitute for medical treatment. It can however, be complementary to the medical treatment. Continue with wise eating, appropriate level of exercises, and medical treatment. This is to encourage you to participate more actively in your treatment. When you participate in your own treatment, you feel you are in control of some things rather than feeling helpless against everything. Mind-body medicine helps you to use your natural resources to strengthen the healing process. You have nothing to lose, in fact by doing so you feel better about yourself, more involved, and more active.

Ø Ø Ø

10. WELLNESS STRATEGIES:
First, Be Happy,
Even If Everyone's Idea Of Happiness
Is Different.

What makes you happy? One might be surprised to find that success, money, health, youth and good looks, and education are not on the top of the list of things that make people happy even though it helps.

Are you ready for this? (4,5,6) People identify "close relationships" and the ability to practice appreciation and love as the number one source of happiness. The runner up is a "happy marriage". Number three is "religious faith"; no matter what religion or what denomination, as long as it is religious faith. The least happy people are those who are in unhappy marriages. Happiest are those who feel that their partners are not just their partners but their "best friend", as well.

Researchers tell us that people normally entertain "predominantly positive emotions" for about seventy-five percent of the time and "predominately unpleasant emotions" for about twenty-five percent of the time. If the time spent between the pleasant and unpleasant emotions is in a ratio of three to one, for example, three hours of pleasant emotions to one hour of unpleasantness, a person is likely to maintain an overall feeling of happiness.

Since we have sixteen waking hours in a day, we should be spending about twelve hours a day with positive thoughts and feelings and not more than four hours with negative thoughts and feelings. Incidentally, the quality of your sleep is also determined by the quality of your thoughts and feelings during the waking hours.

Our thoughts also influence our mood. Talking about troubles has a positive effect on mood. Thinking about troubles has a negative effect on mood. What it boils down to is this: Talking about bad things is not as bad as is thinking about bad things.

Let us really watch our thinking because a lot of times, we are not aware when we are thinking and what we are thinking. We are just thinking.

Happiness is a little bit external and a lot more internal. How much happiness one will have in one's life depends, largely, on one's temperament and attitude. Some are born happy, smiley, and easy to please. Some are born unhappy, whiny, and difficult to please.

Compared to the children with "difficult temperament, " happy-to-be children smile more, are easily comforted, and when they get upset, their crying, kicking, and fussing does not last as long. They tend to be more content. Temperament plays a role in determining whether you spend more time of your life being happy or unhappy.

Our attitudes also contribute to the making of our happiness. Abraham Lincoln once said that people can be as happy or unhappy as they make up their mind to be. Take the example of a positive mental attitude.

When you are upset, positive mental attitude helps you to recover faster and negative emotions do not reach the extremes. Anticipating positive outcomes create hope and optimism. As moments of unhappiness decrease, moments of happiness increase. Why is happiness so elusive? It is so because we believe that "THINGS " rather than "THOUGHTS " make us happy. Therefore, we run after or wait for things to make us happy.

For example, "When I get a bigger house, or that sports car, or that million dollars, I'll be happy". We remain unhappy while we wait for these things to happen. You know they do not happen soon enough. When we finally get the desired thing, we soon get used to it and it does not offer us the same happiness that it once did.

Monetary happiness is like a fever and a lot of people who have obtained a sudden major windfall, note that their happiness shoots up like the temperature in a thermometer on a hot day in July. However, the mercury soon cools down as the money heat wave moves into winter. Usually, within a year these people are only marginally happier than they were before the "gold rush".

Windfalls lose their impact over time because we get used to them. If happiness is what you are after, then why not make up your mind to be happy. Make a deliberate effort to be happy. Do not wait for things to happen in order to make you happy. On the other hand, things may happen when you do whatever you do, happily!

You have no double blind prospective or retrospective studies from any peer reviewed unbiased journal in the world to contradict any information that I have provided to my fellow human beings. The bottomline is – IT WORKS! IT IS SAFE. TRY IT TO SEE IF IT WORKS FOR YOU.

79

These are simply guidelines to help you understand how to use safe natural energy products and technologies, along with balanced nutrition, supplements, and exercise to build a happier, better quality of life for human beings in general and to help them incorporate the best and most simplistic training methods available that are most suitable for achieving maximum martial arts training and maximum quality of life experiences. For more detailed and practical applications to different physical or mental challenges in everyday living or sports, be sure to read "LIFE FORCE-JUST FOR THE HEALTH OF IT!" I have taken the Action to write this upcoming series of books to inform you about what I have learned in general about traditional as well as complementary medicine before and after my retirement.

The Rest Is Up To You !!!

REFERENCED FOOTNOTES

1)Michael I. Weintraub and Steven P. Cole,(Neuromagnetic treatment of pain in refractory carpal tunnel
    syndrome: An electrophysiological placebo analysis) J.of Back and Musculoskeletal Rehabilitation Vol. 15,
        No.2-3(92000) 77-81.

2) M. Weintraub,(Chronic submaximal magnetic stimulation in peripheral neuropathy: Is there a beneficial
        therapeutic relationship) Amer J. Pain Management 8(1998), 12-16.

3)Carlos Valbona, Carlton Hazelwood and G. Jurida,(Response of pain to static magnetic fields in post
        patients: A double blind pilot study) Arch Phys Med Rehab 78(1997) 1200-1203.

4)Richard Corliss, (Is there a formula for joy) Time Magazine-How Your Mind Can Heal Your Body
        Jan 20, 2003.

5)Dan Baker Ph.D. and Cameron Stauth,(What Happy People Know)Rodale 2003.

6)Martin E. P. Seligman Ph.D.(Authentic Happiness: Using the New Positive Psychology to Realize your Potential for Lasting Fulfillment)The Free Press 2002.

LIFEFORCE BOOK

LIFEFORCE: JUST FOR THE HEALTH OF IT!

A Complete Guide to Total Wellness

END MATERIAL:

Appendix One: Bibliography
Appendix Two: Helping Hands and Resource Guide
Appendix Three: Practical Applications of Natural Energy Products

To Order:

Use your "Pay Pal" account or obtain a free account by clicking onto www.paypal.com and follow the prompts to make payment of $15.95 US to: bewater_beone@yahoo.com

Or send check to : Be Water, Be One
                    6671 Walnutwood Circle
                    Baltimore, Maryland 21212 USA